WILDERNESS FIR

THE ULTIMATE BEGINNER'S GUIDE ON HOW TO TREAT INJURIES, CURE INFECTIONS, AND SAVE LIVES IN A LIFE OR DEATH SURVIVAL SITUATION

Bartholomew Rommel

© 2016

Table of Contents

INTRODUCTION

Hey there, thank you for downloading this book, "Wilderness First Aid: the Ultimate Beginner's Guide On How to Treat Injuries, Cure Infections, and Save Lives in a Life or Death Survival Situation."

First aid is defined as the rapid treatment of a person who has become the victim of either an injury or an illness, as a temporary solution until proper medical aid arrives. Even though first aid is generally not intended to be the end solution to healing a person, it can save their life and ensure a faster recovery.

Examples of conditions that will most certainly require first aid include poisoning, stroke, heart attacks, bleeding, frostbite, shock, burns, stings, fainting, broken bones, and difficulty breathing.

In this book, we will cover many different first aid topics in detail with an emphasis on how you can complete the first aid in a survival situation with limited or natural resources. The information that you will learn here will likely be some of the most important information that you ever learn in your life because it can save your life or that of another person, including someone who you care for deeply.

The different first aid topics that we will cover in this book include:

- The Basics of First Aid

- Performing CPR

- Personal Hygiene

- Carrying a Wounded Person

- Treating Sunstroke, Hypothermia, and Dehydration

- Treating an Open Wound

- Treating Scrapes for Infections

- Splinting a Broken Limb

- Treating a Leg Fracture

- Recognizing and Using Wild Medicinal Plants

- Treating a Bullet Wound

- Treating a Knife Wound

- Treating a Bite

- Disease Control

Without any further ado, let's begin!

Chapter One – Principles of Giving First Aid

First aid, in its simplest form, is defined as the process of addressing the medical needs of a person who has either been physically injured or has been the victim of another form of medical emergency such as difficulty breathing, an allergic reaction, a heart attack, an infection, etc.

Basic first aid treatment requires you to assess the condition of the patient, whether it be yourself or someone else, and then correct the problem by using proper treatment. This applies to all kinds of medical needs ranging from something as simple as a small scrape to a more serious injury such as a broken bone.

When you're out in the wilderness and an injury happens to you or a member in your group, you'll be away from any kind of professional medical help and will therefore need to give the first aid yourself. Even though it is no doubt an intimidating and stressful task, first aid skills enable you to provide a temporary solution to the victim to keep them alive until you do reach professional medical help. Knowing about basic first aid procedures and being able to apply them is ultimately what can make the difference between life and death in a survival situation.

In this chapter, we will cover the five fundamental principles of giving wilderness first aid and how you can use them even while under stress:

PRINCIPLE #1 – PRESERVE THE LIFE OF EVERYONE INVOLVED

The ultimate goal of giving first aid is to preserve the life of the victim, and that's why this is our first principle of giving first aid. Preserving life also isn't just limited to the victim; it also includes you and anyone else in your group.

As you approach the victim, do so quickly but also use that time to look around the area and determine if anyone else is a victim or if anyone is in immediate danger. For example, if you come across a car accident and there's a person lying wounded on the road, as you run towards them you should look around to observe if anyone else has been injured in the accident. It's also important that you keep yourself out of harm's way, so keep your eyes and ears open for anything that presents itself as a major threat to you. After all, you're no good to the injured person if you're injured or killed in the process of trying to help them.

PRINCIPLE #2 – EVALUATE THE PATIENT BEFORE TREATING THEM

One reason why it's important to know proper first aid techniques is because even though you may have the right intentions of helping an injured victim, if you don't know what you're doing you could potentially make their wounds or injures worse in the process of trying to help them.

Fortunately, you can ensure that you don't make the victim's pain or injury worse by systematically evaluating them before prescribing treatment. For example, you may see the patient bleeding and decide to immediately give treatment to the best of your ability. But you haven't evaluated them yet. Sure, you see that they are bleeding, but do you know where the bleeding is coming from? Do you know what caused the bleeding? Have you asked the patient how significant the pain is and if they are hurting anywhere else?
These are just a handful of questions that you will need answered before you begin giving treatment, and it's important that you have them answered quickly so you don't begin giving treatment too late.

The best way to evaluate a patient is to examine their head and then work your way down all the way to their toes. Only then will you be able to identify all injuries on the patient and the source of each one. In addition, if at all possible, avoid moving the patient until you have applied the treatments.

PRINCIPLE #3 – KEEP THE VICTIM'S AIRWAY OPEN

It's absolutely essential that the victim's airway be open so they can breathe properly. To check if the airway is open, confirm if they are breathing. If the patient is not breathing, then you'll need to intervene so they can. Open their jaw while being careful to not disturb the rest of the head or the spine; doing so can only cause the trauma to be worse. If there is an object inside the patient's mouth or throat that is inhibiting their airway, you must remove it. If the victim vomits as a result of your intervention, roll them onto their side so it can drain.

PRINCIPLE #4 – KEEP THE PATIENT BREATHING

You may think that this principle is essentially the same as the last one, but the reality is that just because the victim's airway is open doesn't mean they are automatically breathing. Fortunately, there are a variety of different methods you can use to decide if the patient is indeed breathing.

You can tell if the patient is or isn't breathing based on their color, movement in their chest, and listening for air movement from their mouth. If the patient is not breathing, the best solution is CPR and the mouth-to-mouth technique. Perform thirty chest compressions at a time, and in between each set, place your mouth over that of the patient and breathe slowly with much volume. The faster or shorter your breaths are, the less likely the air will reach the patient's lungs.

PRINCIPLE #5 – KEEP THE VICTIM'S BLOOD CIRCULATING

The last principle of first aid is to keep the victim's blood circulating. The factors for determining the status of their circulation is the color of their skin (purple or blue colored skin indicates disturbed or nonexistent circulation), their pulse (a pulse above one hundred is bad), and how long it takes their finger to go from white to normal pink after squeezing it (more than three seconds should cause concern for you).

Bleeding is a major cause of death in medical situations, particularly with trauma. If the patient is bleeding, you have to stop it. Apply pressure to the source of the bleeding either with a sterile cloth or medical gloves. If bleeding continues, you should apply a tourniquet above the wound.

Chapter Two – Personal Hygiene

Many survival situations that may require first aid can be avoided just by using proper personal hygiene techniques.

Something that many people tend to neglect when it comes to survival is grooming. The reason why grooming is neglected in a survival situation is because people have other priorities that they believe require more immediate attention. It's completely understandable if water, food, warmth/shelter, and security are your top priorities in a survival situation. Each of those things is vitally important in its own right.

But you have to keep in mind that grooming can and will significantly boost your chances of making it out alive in ANY survival situation. Basic grooming procedures will keep away deadly bacteria and diseases that can infect your body and contaminate your water. Plain and simple, the cleaner you are in a survival situation, the higher chance you will have at making it out alive and in good health.

Here are the basic principles of grooming that will ensure you and your family can avoid deadly infections and diseases in your quest for survival:

WASH YOUR HANDS

This is perhaps the most basic personal hygiene rule but it's still very important. You should always wash your hands in a survival situation or disaster scenario after handling anything that possibly carries bacteria, after using the bathroom, and before you handle food and water. If you don't have soap and a little water available to wash your hands, you can always use hand sanitizer.

CLEAN YOUR CLOTHES

Your clothing covers your entire body, including your largest organ: your skin. If your clothes become infested with parasites, your chances of developing a skin infection go up dramatically and this is something you absolutely must avoid. Obviously you most likely won't have a working washing machine in a survival situation, but you can keep your clothes clean by keeping them dry, cleaning them with soap and water on a regular basis, and swapping out different articles of clothing each day. It's especially important to swap out your socks regularly as a defense against gangrene.

CLEAN YOUR HAIR

If your hair goes unattended, it can easily become infested with bacteria and parasites that are one of the biggest causes of disease and infection in a survival scenario. The best defenses against this will be to trim your hair when it begins to grow long, to keep it combed (include a comb in your survival kit), and to clean it with soap or shampoo on a daily basis. Even washing your hair with just warm, clean water each morning will help.

ORAL HYGIENE

You'll want to clean your teeth at least once every day in order to ensure that they remain completely free of harmful oral bacteria. If you don't have your toothbrush or toothpaste with you, a natural alternative is a chewing stick. Separate the fiber on the stick by chewing on both ends and then use that to brush your teeth. You can also rub your teeth clean with some cloth wrapped around your fingers or even salt on your finger tip. It may not seem like much, but it can certainly go a long way to ensure that your teeth are taken care of.

CLEAN YOUR FEET

When you don't have access to a motorized vehicle or a bicycle, your feet are literally the only way you can transport yourself from place to place (assuming you're not a fan of crawling). This is why it's absolutely imperative that your feet remain in top condition throughout your survival endeavor. Swap out your socks on a daily basis and have the old pair dry out before putting them on the next day. This will help to prevent gangrene. Make sure that your toe nails remain short, and rub your feet with your hands at the end of each day to relax them. Soak your feet in a bucket or wrap them in a bandana of hot water and use soap if you have it. Make it a habit to check your shoes for any debris that gets in there and remove them immediately.

PURIFYING WATER

Purifying water is exceptionally important in order to prevent serious illness. In fact, water purification is one of the biggest safety procedures when it comes to survival. Make it a habit to clean your drinking water via filtration, purification tablets, or boiling (or better yet, a combination of those) to confirm that it is absolutely safe to drink before you even think of drinking a drop of it. As another safety precaution, it is also a good idea to avoid collecting any water from questionable sources. Avoid taking water downstream of animal feces or near an area of known chemical contamination, for examples.

PROPER WASTE DISPOSAL

Probably the most popular method of proper human waste disposal in a survival situation is to dig a cat hole. This is a hole that is between six inches to one foot deep and about half as wide. After using the cat hole, fill it back up with the dirt that you just removed in order to ensure that the feces are completely covered.

Always dig your cat holes a minimum of two hundred feet away from your camp, any other resources you have such as a food storage area, and especially from a water source such as a lake or river. Use toilet paper, napkins, paper towels, notebook paper, or whatever you have available; using plants as toilet paper should be a last resort and only use plants that you are highly familiar with. Finally, with no exceptions, always wash your hands either with soap and warm water or hand sanitizer after using the bathroom.

PERSONAL HYGIENE ITEMS TO HAVE IN YOUR SURVIVAL KIT

Here is a list of personal hygiene items that you would be wise to include in your survival kit or bug out bag, in alphabetical order:

- Baking Soda
- Bandana
- Comb
- Cotton Swab
- Deodorant
- Hand Sanitizer
- Nail File
- Paper Towels
- Razor
- Shampoo
- Soap
- Toilet Paper
- Toothbrush
- Toothpaste
- Towel
- Wet Wipes

Almost everyone agrees that personal hygiene is important in our daily lives, but significantly fewer people rank it as high of importance as finding water, building fire and shelter, or taking security measures in a survival situation or in a disaster scenario.

But here's the truth: infections and diseases can be deadly in a survival situation, especially in a community that has been already damaged by a disaster. You don't need to look any further than the earthquake disaster in Haiti, for example, to see how quick diseases can spread and how many lives they can claim.

But just because you don't have running water or soap and shampoo doesn't mean that you can't take simple personal hygiene and sanitation measures. In this article, we will explore how you can keep yourself clean in a survival or disaster scenario by making homemade personal hygiene items.

MAKING YOUR OWN SOAP FOR PERSONAL HYGIENE

The principles of how soap works are simple: it take particles that cannot be dissolved in water (insoluble) and makes it so that they can be dissolved in water (soluble).

Examples of particles that are insoluble include oil, grease, grime, and dirt that is mixed in with any of those previous three things.

If grease and/or oil mixed with dirt get on your hands and you try to wash them off with water only, nothing will happen. But soap will mix with the water and carry those greases and oils away. This is why soap can truly make your hands 'clean,' and it's also why it's important to have and use soap in a survival situation.

If you don't have any soap already with you, you're not out of luck. Making soap is just as simple as understanding how soap works itself. For example, you can make a very effective soap out of nothing more than animal fat and ash from wood:

1. Take two containers of different sizes, and punch a hole through the smaller one
2. Fill one inch of the smaller container up with a layer of gravel
3. Fill a layer of sand over the layer of gravel
4. Fill the rest of your container with ash
5. Place the smaller container inside of the larger container
6. Pour water through the small container, slowly but steadily, so that it comes out in a brown/grey color in the second container
7. Boil the brown/grey water in your second container until half of it is evaporated
8. Add at least one cup of animal fat to this mixture and continue to boil it for thirty minutes (the fat must be free of all blood and meat, or else the soap will spoil)
9. Pour the mixture into your desired shape of molds
10. Give the molds two days to dry, and then remove the resulting soap
11. Cut the soap into your desired sizes and store in a well-ventilated area

MAKING YOUR OWN DEODORANT FOR PERSONAL HYGIENE

While soap can make you clean, it can't always remove your body of the stench of body odor. This is where deodorant comes into play, and not only can it make you smell better, but it can also help prevent bacteria from growing on your underarms.

To make your own deodorant for personal hygiene, you will need baking soda (something that should probably be in your survival kit), corn starch, coconut oil, and essential oils (such as cinnamon, ginger, lavender, peppermint, spearmint, etc).

You can make DIY deodorant using the following process:

1. Mix your baking soda with corn starch, and make sure there are equal parts of each
2. Add a few drops of your essential oil of choice
3. Add at least two tablespoons of coconut oil
4. Mix all of the ingredients together

5. Place the mixture into a container, and allow the container to dry for at least two days to make your deodorant

MAKING YOUR OWN TOOTHPASTE FOR PERSONAL HYGIENE

Keeping your teeth and gums clean is just as important as keeping your skin clean. Not only will dirty and rotting teeth give you an unpleasant bad breath, but it can lead to harmful oral bacteria setting in and causing problems.

Did you know that you can make an effective survival toothpaste with nothing more than baking soda and some warm water? There's definitely a reason why baking soda is the primary ingredient in almost all commercial toothpastes. It's an extremely simple process to make too: you literally only have to mix in enough baking soda with your water until a paste forms.

It won't taste the same as commercial toothpaste, to say the least, but this DIY toothpaste will definitely keep your teeth and gums clean, and that's what matters. This is also one more reason why you should include some baking soda in your survival kit.

Chapter Three – Disease Control

Epidemiology is defined as a branch of medicine dealing with the distribution and the control of infections and diseases. In the post-modern age we live in today, we have become almost entirely dependent on modern day drugs. The good thing about these drugs, specifically in the form of anti-viral medicine and antibiotics, is that they have helped to get rid of infections and diseases in many parts of the world.

The bad news is that once these drugs are no longer used, the diseases and infections will very likely return. In the event of a large scale and long term disaster, the ability to manufacture these drugs will become inhibited if not stopped entirely. Epidemiology is all about how we can prevent these diseases from occurring in such a scenario.

Medical preparedness doesn't mean that you have to become a medical professional or an expert by any means; it simply means that you take responsibility upon yourself to learn various medical techniques and sanitation procedures, and find out how you can apply them to stop the invasion of infections in your family or survival group.

Before we learn more about epidemiology, let's get an understanding of what causes infections and diseases to happen in the first place.

WHAT CAUSES INFECTIONS AND DISEASES?

The chief cause of infections and diseases come from pathogens, which are harmful microbes in the form of germs, viruses, bacteria, and protozoa. Viruses in particular are able to reproduce at alarmingly high rates, while protozoa are most often caught from water and invade the body when the infected water is consumed.

Pathogens in general are carried to people by vectors, which are defined as other people or animals who carry a disease and transmit it to other people. One example of a vector would be a mosquito that carries malaria, for example.

BASIC PREVENTATIVE TECHNIQUES FOR INFECTIONS AND DISEASES

For the rest of this article, we will learn some basic preventative techniques you can use in regards to both your personal health and the general sanitation of an area that will keep infections and diseases away. The stricter the hygiene standards you set for your group are (and the more rigorously enforced they are), the healthier your group will be.

- Washing Hands

  - Regular and proper hand washing is critical when it comes to epidemiology. Always lather your hands in soap first, making sure that all parts of the hand including the palms, back of the hand, and in between the fingers are lathered. Then, run your hands under warm water for a minimum of thirty seconds and rub vigorously.

  - Hand washing should be completed at regular times in the day, such as after going to the bathroom, before eating, and before and after treating a patient.

- Respiratory Hygiene

  - Equally as important as washing hands is respiratory hygiene, and it especially applies to those who in your group who are coughing and sneezing often. Always cover the mouth and nose completely with a tissue when making a cough or a sneeze, and wash your hands afterwards using the above procedures.

- If you lack tissues, napkins, handkerchiefs, or anything of the sort, use either your inner elbow or upper arm to cough and sneeze. NEVER cough or sneeze into your hands.

- If coughing and sneezing persists with someone in their group, have them wear an N95 mask throughout the day, and if possible keep them a short distance away from the rest of the group. If you don't have N95 masks with you, you can make do with bandanas or old shirts.

- Clean Water

  - We noted before that water is the primary avenue for protozoa to infect a group. Therefore all water used by your group, for drinking, cleaning, and personal hygiene purposes, must be clean and sterile before you even think of using it for those purposes.

  - There are many different ways that you can clean water. Boiling water for at least thirty minutes is the most surefire way of killing all harmful organisms and chemicals in the water. You can also sterilize the water by running it through large water filters, and dropping at least two iodine purification tablets in for thirty minutes. Better yet, use a combination of these methods to ensure that your water is clean.

- Clean Food

  - Organisms that cause diseases can be present on the outside parts of certain kinds of foods, including vegetables and fruits. Another use you can have for water is to rinse food before cooking it. Again, make sure that your water has been sterilized via the above methods before using it to rinse food.

  - When cooking meats, it's imperative that you cook at high enough temperatures so you can confirm that any harmful bacteria have been eliminated. A temperature of at least one hundred and sixty five degrees Fahrenheit is a good rule of thumb to follow for cooking any kind of meats.

- Human Waste Disposal

  - One of the biggest causes of the spreads of infections and diseases is improper disposal of human waste. A good use for water that is not safe for drinking is to pour it into the toilet after using it. Pouring at least two gallons of water into the toilet will activate the siphoning mechanism, and it will flush even without running water.

- Digging a cat hole at least six inches deep and wide and then refilling it up with dirt after use is the best way to dispose of human waste for individuals, but for groups, you should dig a trench that everybody can use. This trench should be a minimum of four feet deep, fifteen feet long, and one foot wide. Use the dirt you removed and a shovel to cover up the excrement. Once the dirt has reached one foot, fill it all the way back up and abandon the trench and re-dig a new one. Each trench must be a minimum of two hundred feet away from your camp and from any water sources. It's also best that the trench be out in the sunlight since the excrement will decompose faster under the sun.

- Caring for the Sick

  - You should have a sick room in your camp that is dedicated to providing space for those who are ill. You should have minimal furniture in the sick room; cots, chairs, and a table is all that is needed. Avoid fabric for flooring, and make sure that the room receives plenty of ventilation.

  - Your sick room should be on the other side of camp from the kitchen and the eating area, and it must have a door and closed windows so it can be shut off from the rest of the camp if necessary. Keep plenty of water, soap, and alcohol in the sick room.

  - The only person who should be allowed in the sick room, other than those who are sick, is your medic. The medic should wear medical gloves and an N95 mask at all times that they are in the sick room, and they must wash their hands before and after treating patients.

  - Routinely disinfect the sick room, especially the work surfaces and furniture, with a bleach solution or baking soda.

Chapter Four – Heatstroke, Hypothermia, and Dehydration

Sunstroke, hypothermia, and dehydration together are among the biggest killers in survival situations. If you're ever stranded out in the wilderness and trying to find your way back to civilization, you cannot let any one of these things slow you down or stop you entirely. In this chapter, we will learn how you can prevent sunstroke, hypothermia, and dehydration from happening, and then also how you can treat them if they do occur.

We will begin with sunstroke:

SUNSTROKE:

Sunstroke, also known as heatstroke, is classified by almost all medical professionals a form of medical emergency and is worst type of heat injury that you can sustain. The reason why sunstroke is so dangerous is because it damages your brains and your internal organs. Older people tend to be more susceptible to it, but even young and athletic people are not invulnerable to it.

Sunstroke will begin as another similar but less severe illness such as heat exhaustion, fainting, heat cramps, or anything related that develops from extended exposure to excessively high temperatures and dehydration. If any one of these illnesses goes without treatment and becomes worse, it can slowly turn into sunstroke. For this reason, immediately seek shade and drink plenty of water if you've fainted as a result of heat or are feeling exhausted from the heat. If you do this, it can hopefully stop the illness from developing into sunstroke.

Officially, sunstroke is defined as a core body temperature of greater than one hundred and five degrees Fahrenheit. Symptoms of sunstroke include seizures, lowered cognitive function, being disoriented, vomiting, and lack of consciousness.

Treating sunstroke is largely dependent on the specific symptoms that you develop. In many instances, you can treat yourself simply by moving to a shaded area, applying a bandana soaked in cool water over your forehead and skin, and drinking plenty of cool water. These things will help return your body to a cool state. If you have access to a stream or lake, immerse your entire body into the water to accelerate the cooling. Drinking a mixture of water, salt, and sugar can also do much to cool you down.

Your neck, back, armpits, and groin have the most blood vessels in your body, so you'll want to focus applying cool water to those areas so that you can cool down faster.

HYPOTHERMIA

Hypothermia is defined as the core temperature in the body dropping to below ninety five degrees Fahrenheit. The initial symptoms of hypothermia include excessive shivering, which is an attempt by your body to decrease the temperature, clumsiness, slow speech, excessive drowsiness, an accelerating heart rate, and shallow breathing.

The scary thing about hypothermia is that it can set in quickly, so you'll need to act quickly to turn it around too.

If you start to become cold and shiver excessively, sitting next to a fire or performing exercises such as jumping jacks are two of the most important things you can do to warm yourself up. But even if the hypothermia sets in anyway, hope is not lost.

The first thing to do once hypothermia sets in is to find shelter very quickly. The purpose of shelter is to form a barrier between the victim (either you or someone else) and the outside elements. If you don't have a tarp or a space blanket with you to do this, then a large tree or an overhanging rock will suffice.

The next thing you must do is to remove any wet clothes that are on you. Rain is one of the most common ways for hypothermia to set in, but sweating on a cold day can also be a cause behind it. Any clothes that become wet as a result will only pull heat out of the body, which makes the hypothermia worse. Remove the wet clothes and replace them with the dry ones if you have them.

The next step is to warm up the body. If you have sleeping bags, blankets, or ponchos, wrap the victim or yourself up in them. Then, you'll need to bring in more warmth into the shelter to warm the body externally. There are three viable ways to accomplish this: have someone lie down next to the victim to share body heat, fill up a bladder with warm water and then place it between the person and their sleeping bag or blanket, or light a fire and lie down next to it.

Now, you'll need to warm the body internally. The best way to warm the body internally, hands down, is to slowly but steadily drink warm liquids. If you get a fire going, you can heat some water over it and then have the victim drink it. With the body now being warmed from the outside and the inside, the hypothermia can be reversed.

DEHYDRATION

Last but not least, we'll talk about how you can treat dehydration. Dehydration is defined as the excessive loss of moisture or water from the body, to the point that metabolic processes are disturbed which is the result of a significant restriction on the intake of water. You should never decide to drink water purely on thirst. Many people can become accustomed to not drinking while thirsty, but then suffer from dehydration later.

When you lost over five percent of your body water, you become anorexic and can sustain heavy migraine headaches. When you lost ten percent of your body water, you will feel excessively dizzy and light headed, and will likely need help getting rehydrated. Losing over fifteen percent of your body water is dangerous and could claim your life.

Obviously the best prevention to stop dehydration from occurring in the first place is to drink plenty of water. Just taking a small sip every ten to fifteen minutes gives your body the fluids it needs to operate normally.

If you do become dehydrated, immediately stop what you are doing so you don't exert the body any further. You'll then need to focus entirely on replenishing your body with water. Fortunately, rehydrating yourself is practically painless. Wrap a bandana soaked in cool water around your head and drink as much water as you can, but rather than drinking an entire bottle all at once, instead drink the water slowly yet steadily. The reason why is because you can have more difficulty drinking while dehydrated, but drinking the water slowly can be easier to gulp. You can also immerse your entire body in a pool or stream of water, but don't drink directly from the source until you've purified or filtered it.

When you are found and get to a hospital, the doctors can then treat any remaining symptoms.

Chapter Five – Performing CPR

CPR, which stands for cardiopulmonary resuscitation, is a medical emergency procedure that is used to preserve the function of the brain until more medical attention is undertaken to restore proper breathing and circulation. CPR is performed on those who are unresponsive and are either not breathing properly or aren't breathing at all.

If this happens to someone in your group while out in the wilderness and away from professional medical attention, then it's up to you to perform CPR to try and save their life.

Here is a step-by-step process for performing CPR:

STEP #1 – CHECK FOR DANGER

You don't want to put yourself in immediate danger when administering CPR to someone. Performing CPR in the middle of a busy road or near a forest fire is the last place you want to do it in. If danger is present you should try to neutralize it, but if you can't, then move the victim by quickly but carefully dragging them to safety.

STEP #2 – ASSESS THE VICTIM AND CHECK THEIR CONSCIOUSNESS

Tap the victim and ask if they are okay, and place your ears next to their mouth to check for breathing. If they respond and are breathing, then it means that they are conscious and you won't need to perform CPR. You can then re-assess the victim and decide what other kind of medical attention is required.

But if the victim does not respond and isn't breathing, you'll need to proceed with the rest of the steps.

STEP #3 – OPEN THE VICTIM'S AIRWAY

If the airway to the victim is blocked or obstructed, then CPR will be useless. This is why it's important for you to confirm that the victim's airway is open before you begin performing chest compressions.

Tilt the victim's head back by lifting their chin and pressing back on their forehead with two fingers on both the chin and the forehead. If a neck injury is present, avoid this technique and pull the jaw forward. Otherwise, go with this technique.

Carefully examine the airway for obstacles by pressing your forefinger and thumb on each cheek and peering inside. Remove any obstacles that you can see with your fingers. If you cannot remove the obstacles with your fingers, use the abdominal thrust method. Once the obstacles, if any, are removed you should immediately proceed with the next step.

STEP #4 – ROLL THE VICTIM ONTO THEIR BACK

Roll the victim flat onto their back if they aren't already. They should be flat as they can be and you'll want to straighten out their limbs as well. Confirm that their airway is still open all the way. Do this quickly so you can get right to the chest compressions as soon as possible.

STEP #5 – POSITION YOURSELF FOR CHEST COMPRESSIONS

This next step is critical, so pay close attention. Place the heel of your dominant hand directly on the breastbone of the victim, and right between their nipples.

Take your non-dominant hand and place it on top of your first hand. Both hands must have the palms facing down, and the fingers should be interlocked for extra security.

Your body should be held right over your hands, to ensure that your elbows are almost locked and that your arms are rigid. This position also enables you to utilize the strength from your upper body to push.

STEP #6 – PERFORM CHEST COMPRESSIONS

This next step is also critical. Once you've positioned yourself to perform the chest compressions, it's immediately time to begin performing the compressions yourself.

For each compression, you'll want to push both of your hands down over the breastbone by at least two inches and at about one hundred beats a minute. You want your compressions to be fast rather than slow, and remember to use your upper body strength meaning your body must be held directly over your arms throughout the process.

Complete a set of thirty chest compressions in this manner, and then pause for a maximum of ten seconds before resuming (a pause of around five seconds would be better). Use this time to again put your ear over their mouth to check for breathing, and then resume if they are not.

STEP #7 – RESCUE BREATHS

Rescue breaths were once considered a necessary part of standard operation for performing CPR, but according to the American Heart Association they are no longer necessary because the chest compressions are far more effective. However, you can still perform a maximum of two rescue breaths in the middle of each pause if you feel confident in that it would help the victim.

Confirm that the airway of the victim is still open and then pinch their nose shut with two fingers. Seal your mouth over the mouth of the victim and exhale two deep breaths of one second each.

When your breath goes in, you will notice the victim's chest rising. This is a confirmation that your breaths have reached the lungs of the victim.

STEP #8 – MORE CHEST COMPRESSIONS

After each pause and quickly checking the victim for breathing (and performing rescue breaths if you feel it is necessary), immediately perform another set of thirty chest compressions in the same manner as before.

After completing a cycle of five sets of thirty chest compressions, tap the victim and check for any signs of life. Tap them and ask if they are okay and listen for breathing.

If you receive no response, continue performing CPR until you are too exhausted, until medical help arrives, or until the victim begins showing signs of life.

STEP #9 – STABILIZE THE VICTIM INTO A RECOVERY POSITION

Wait to stabilize the victim until after their breathing has returned to the point that they are breathing comfortably without any aid.

Raise one of their knees so that one leg is bent upwards and the other is straight. Roll the victim onto the side of their straight leg; the bent knee on the other leg ensures that they don't fall onto their abdomen. When rolling the victim onto their side, do so by positioning your hand on the opposite shoulder of their straight leg. Your other hand should be placed on the edge of the hip of the bent leg.

This position is known as the recovery position and permits the victim to breathe easily. It also stops saliva from gathering in the throat that would inhibit their breathing.

Give the victim some time to regain complete control over their breathing and to regain full consciousness. Ask how they are feeling and go from there, and seek professional medical help for further attention as soon as possible.

Chapter Six – Treating Scrapes

Before the age of modern medications and technology, one of the biggest killers of man was infection. Even the smallest cut can cause an infection, so it cannot be overstated how important it is for any kind of an injury sustained in a survival situation to receive immediate and careful attention, especially since you likely don't have access to modern medicines and technologies.

To put this into perspective, if you trip and fall and receive a scrape to your knee or elbow, it may seem like nothing more than an annoyance now, but if it goes long enough without treatment a serious life-threatening infection could potentially set in. That's why it's so important for you to immediately tend to any kind of a minor scrape that you or anyone in your survival group receives. The good news is that if you do tend to your scrape and keep it under management, you stand a much greater chance of survival.

In this chapter, we will cover how you can treat scrapes for infections, starting with an understanding of how an open would stands a significant chance of becoming infected in the first place.

HOW CAN A SIMPLE SCRAPE BECOME INFECTED?

The reason why open wounds are weak points for infection is because the protective barrier of skin is ripped open and the flesh underneath is exposed. The inside parts of your body are almost completely unprotected to bacteria and pathogens.

Your body can receive these bacteria from a number of different ways. They can come from dirt or outside debris that gets into the wound, from a knife or another sharp object that caused the injury, or even from floating around in the air and landing on the wound. It's possible for the deadliest of bacteria to get into the smallest of wounds, which is why even a seemingly harmless scrape must be treated.

HOW CAN YOU TELL IF YOUR SCRAPE IS INFECTED?

You can generally tell if your scrape has become infected with something based on the following systems:

- Discoloration on the open flesh: even a slight discoloration such as a slightly darker redness can be a sign of infection.

- Fever: a fever is the result of the body's natural reaction to increasing its inside temperature to try and kill the bacteria.

- Inflammation: this is also a natural response of the body to an infection, where it slows blood flow to the affected area and causes that area to swell.

- Pus: that yellow/green pus that can come out of an open would is an attempt by the body to collect the bacteria; the pus will need to be drained immediately so that it carries much of the bacteria with it.

It's hard to think that the smallest scrape on your knee can lead to a disease as serious as gangrene, but it can happen. That's why you can never be too careful.

Next, we'll discuss how you can treat a scrape, followed with a discussion on how you can treat an infection that results from that scrape.

TREATING THE SCRAPE

If an open wound is small enough, it will not need stitches and can heal easily on its own. You'd actually be amazed at how effective the human body is at healing on its own. A scrape definitely falls into the category of a small wound, or at least the overwhelming majority of 'scrapes' do, so closing the wound via suturing is not necessary for treatment here.

The best way to treat the scrape will be to clean it and then dress/bandage it. A mix of clean water with hydrogen peroxide or alcohol works the best, but if you lack either of these, then just clean water will work. Never clean a scrape or open wound of any kind with dirty water, because it can potentially cause more outside debris or bacteria to get into the wound, which only increases the odds of infection. Boil, purify, and/or filter your water before using it for treating a scrape.

Once you've flushed out the wound with open water, it's time to dress it. If the scrape is quite small, then only a simple bandage out of your first aid kit will be enough to keep it from getting infected by your environment. For a larger scrape, however, you'll need something like sterile gauze pads, bandanas, or cloths.

Dampen your first gauze pad or cloth in water and then set this directly over the scrape. This gauze pad or cloth must be completely clean to prevent infection, so a dirty rag you have in your survival pack won't work.

Then, apply a dry cloth around the first. Ideally, this dry cloth should be a little larger than the first cloth, and it must also be clean. Secure the cloth either by tying or taping it. The entire scrape must be completely covered.

TREATING AN INFECTION

Check on your scrape at least once or twice every day, and look for visible signs of infection such as discoloration. If the scrape does not heal in a few days, apply antibiotic treatment if you have it, or re-clean and re-dress the wound. Monitoring your wound is imperative for the next few days, and you should avoid overexertion and get plenty of rest so that your body has the best chance of avoiding or overcoming any kind of an infection.

If treated right, your wound will heal naturally and any kind of an infection that develops will be overcome. If the scrape becomes worse and dead flesh appears, you'll need to open the wound up and expose it to the flies for at least a day. Wait for the maggots to eat the dead flesh before flushing them out with water and then redressing the wound; the scrape should heal naturally afterwards. But since it's a simple scrape, there likely won't be a need for this.

Once you make it out to safety, have a medical professional evaluate your scrape and treat any remaining symptoms that you have.

Chapter Seven – Open Wounds

While an open wound certainly provides the challenge of having to deal with the loss of blood and damage to tissue, the real danger is that the wound could become infected. The flesh could have come into contact with dirty skin or clothing, bacteria could be in the wound that hasn't been removed, or foreign debris could get into the wound and contaminate it.

An open wound should never, under any circumstances, go without treatment in a survival situation (or ever, for that matter). First, let's outline and discuss the different kinds of open wounds, and then we'll go into a step-by-step process for how you can treat these wounds and prevent an infection from setting in.

TYPES OF OPEN WOUNDS

- Abrasion

    - An abrasion is essentially the same thing as a scrape. It's when the skin rubs against a rough surface, tearing apart the skin and exposing the flesh inside. Bleeding is mostly minimal in comparison to other open wounds, but it still runs the risk of infection and must be treated.

- Avulsion

    - An avulsion is the tearing of both skin and tissue. An example of an avulsion would be a gunshot wound. Avulsions bleed very rapidly so immediate treatment is required.

- Incision

    - An incision is where a knife or another type of sharp object cleanly cuts into the skin and flesh. Incisions are the most bloody of open wounds and furthermore can potentially cause damage to the muscles, tendons, and the internal organs.

- Laceration

  - A laceration is an irregular deep cut or slash in the skin, typically the result of an accident with a knife or another tool. There is a lot of bleeding involved and treatment is immediately required.

- Puncture

  - A puncture is defined as a wound caused by a pointed object such as needle or nail. Punctures rarely bleed much but if the sharp object traveled far enough, the internal organs could be damaged.

HOW TO TREAT AN OPEN WOUND

Now that we've learned about what the main different types of open wounds, let's learn about what you should do should any of these happen to you or somebody in your group.

- Assess the Victim

  - First thing is first in a first aid situation: you have to assess the victim and examine all injuries on the body. Determine the severity of each injury and which one deserves your most immediate attention.

- Stop the Bleeding

  - Next, you need to stop or at least inhibit the bleeding on each open wound. Start with the more serious wounds first, or the ones that are bleeding the most. But rather than wrapping a tourniquet above the open wound, as many people may feel inclined to do, you should stead apply direct pressure over the wound with a barrier between your skin and the wound. This barrier can either come in the form of sterile medical gloves, or it can be a clean bandana or article of clothing.

- If the wound is on a limb, have the victim lay down flat on their back and elevate the limb above their heart. This will stop a lot of blood from traveling to the wounded area and slow the rate of bleeding.

- Clean the Wound

  - Next, you need to clean the wound(s). This step is imperative because a wound that is dirty is ripe for an infection. Once the bleeding stops, remove the dressing that you have set for it and pour some water over the wound at a perpendicular angle. Pour the water slowly, but also steadily enough so that any dirt or foreign matter inside of the wound is flushed out. The water you use should be the cleanest water you have available, since dirty water can only get more contaminants into the wound.

- Dress the Wound

  - Once the wound has stopped bleeding and has been cleaned, it's time to dress it. Don't close, or suture, the wound unless if it won't stop bleeding or won't close on its own after time. Ideally, suturing should be left to a medical professional and dressing the wound is used as a temporary solution until you can get the victim to safety and a hospital.

  - To dress the wound, you'll want to use a moist paid underneath a dry pad. A good example of a makeshift dressing you could use in the wilderness would be a damp gauze pad covered with a dry gauze pad and then secured with tape, or a gauze pad and then a bandana for a larger wound. You want the dressing to completely cover the wound so that no outside contaminants can get inside.

  - Have the victim lay down in a comfortable position with a bandana soaked in water over their forehead. Make sure that they get plenty of rest and have them stay fully hydrated; the best way to assure this is to have them take a small sip of water at least once every ten to fifteen minutes.

  - Check on the dressing at least once every twelve hours. Scan the wound like a hawk for infection, and if the wound has discolored, swollen, or has oozed puss, remove the dressing, clean the wound again, and leave it open for at least a day before redressing.

- Prevent Shock

- Throughout this whole process, you have to maintain blood circulation to the brain of the victim so that shock does not set in. Symptoms of shock include clammy skin, a rapid heartbeat, shallow breathing, and vomiting. If shock sets in, keep the victim wrapped in a blanket next to a fire so that they are warm, keep them fully hydrated, and turn them onto their side when they vomit.

HANDLING INFECTION

It's likely that infection is inevitable with an open wound in a survival situation, but you can minimize this infection with the following steps:

- Give the victim antibiotics (if you have any)
- Place a warm compress over the wound for thirty minutes at a time, at least three times a day
- Use a probe to drain the wound once a day
- Have the victim remain fully hydrated
- Open the wound to flies for at least one day, and then redress it
- Check for maggots, and remove them only once they have killed the dead tissue and before they begin eating the healthy tissue
- Flush the wound with clean water daily

In time, the wound should heal normally and any infections that develop will be small if this method is followed.

It cannot be overstated enough about how learning how to give first aid properly is not only one of the most important survival skills you can learn, but one of the most important life skills you can learn in general. One of the biggest aspects of first aid is suturing, which is defined as stitching together or closing the edges of either a medical incision or an open wound.

Most survival first aid kits have the necessary equipment for suturing, but it's more important that you actually know how to suture a wound then it is to have the actual equipment. Suturing a wound the wrong way can not only cause the victim more pain, but it can also make their wound worse. In this article, we will cover how to suture a wound properly:

STEP #1 – DECIDING TO SUTURE THE WOUND

In general, you should only suture a wound when no other options are viable. The reason why suturing should be a last resort method is because ideally you should clean and bandage a wound and then allow it to heal on its own. You'd be surprised at how proficient the human body is at self-healing when left alone.

But if the wound is not staying together or if the bleeding won't stop, then it's safer to suture the wound rather than simply cleaning and bandaging it. Like we mentioned in our introduction, suturing only works when done the right way, and that's what we're going to learn about next.

STEP #2 – ASSEMBLING YOUR SUTURING EQUIPMENT

Hopefully, you'll have all of the equipment that you need to suture a wound in your first aid kit. Here is a checklist for a complete suturing kit, in alphabetical order:

- Alcohol Prep Wipes
- Clean Water
- Gauze Pads
- Medical Bowl
- Medical Gloves
- Medical Scissors
- Needle
- Needle Driver
- Surgical Probe
- Suture Threads
- Syringe
- Tape
- Tweezers

Keep in mind that there is an extremely wide variety of sizes and types of suturing threads, needles, and so on available on the market. It's wise to include a variety of different sizes in your first aid kit for different wounds. The smaller or more delicate the wound is, then the smaller size of needle and thread you will need.

In addition, make sure that all of your medical tools are clean and sterile before using them. If they are dirty, they can potentially cause an infection to develop in the victim when they come into contact with the wound.

STEP #3 – CLEAN THE WOUND

The third step in suturing a wound is clean the wound first. This is a more critical step than most people realize. Wear medical gloves and always use clean water for this step; contaminated water or an unclean wound are ingredients for an infection setting in, which you definitely don't want. Use a syringe to get the water directly onto the wound, and be careful so you don't cause significantly more pain or make the injury worse. Cleaning the wound also helps to slow down the bleeding if it hasn't been stopped already. The wound should be made as clean as possible before you begin the actual suturing process.

STEP #4 – SUTURING THE WOUND

In very general terms, suturing is simply tying knots over the open wound to help the skin to close. Don't forget that the health of the victim is your top priority, so you don't want to make your knots too tight or complicated so that they only cause more pain, while also not making them too simple or loose so that they don't close the wound properly.

Here is a checklist to run through when actually suturing a wound. As you'll soon see, it's a relatively simple process:

- Observe the wound and definitively confirm that it needs to be sutured rather than simply cleaned and bandaged; again, make sure that your medical gloves are on and that your medical equipment is sterile

- After cleaning the wound from Step #3, confirm that no debris of any kind is present inside the wound; if there is, remove it

- Use your needle driver to grab the needle and then thread it

- Always begin in the center of the wound and then work outward in both directions

- Keep a little bit of space in between each stitch; at least an eighth of an inch is a good rule of thumb

- Once the wound has been stitched, bandage it up with a gauze pad and tape

STEP #5 – PREVENTING AN INFECTION

Keeping the victim healthy after the suture is equally as important as the suturing process itself. The primary goal of this step is to ensure that an infection is avoided at all costs.

Here is a checklist to follow to ensure that the victim recovers properly and that a suture is avoided:

- Change the gauze pads out twice every day and use new tape with each changing

- Check on the condition of the wound and for an infection each time after swapping out the gauze pads

- If the wound does not begin healing after a few days or if you see evidence of an infection, re-open the wound carefully and check for debris inside the wound; carefully re-suture using the process described in Step #4

- Give the victim plenty of food and water and keep them lying down; if a headache sets in, place a bandana soaked in cool water over their forehead and make sure they get plenty of rest

- Get the victim to professional medical help as soon as possible

Chapter Eight – Splinting a Fractured Limb

Even though the wilderness may be the worst place for you to fracture a limb, it's also unfortunately the place where it could be the most likely to happen to you. The reason is because the wild has not exactly been made safe for humans to live in. There are no safety precautions, and hazards are everywhere. This is why thousands of people sustain injuries when out in the wilds each year, and many of those injuries are a broken limb.

It is possible to break practically any bone in your body in the wilderness. However, the vast majority of broken bones that have occurred with those out in the wilderness are either the upper or lower arm, or the upper or lower leg. The most common reason why these bones are broken is because of falls.

If you suffer a broken bone when stranded out in the wilderness, it will certainly be a detriment to you walking out and finding your way back to civilization, but if you know what to do you it won't stop you from surviving. In this article we will cover what is arguably the most important step in treating a broken limb in detail: making a splint.

But first, remember the difference between the two different types of broken bones, which are open fractures and closed fractures. The difference between these two is that in an open fracture, the skin has been ripped open in the process of the bone being broken, and many times the bone will actually protrude out of the skin. Not exactly a pretty thing to think about, but that's what an open fracture is. On the other hand, a closed fracture is where the skin has not torn or where the bone has not penetrated the skin. So if you're splinting a limb with an open fracture, you'll also need to make sure that you dress the open wound as well.

Improvising a splint out of natural materials in the wilderness will require a little creativity on your part, but as long as you know the fundamentals you can do it.

STEP #1 – GATHERING YOUR MATERIALS

Your splints can be made out of anything from an axe handle to a thick walking stick from the forest. What matters is that you need two splints, both of the same or almost the same length and roughly the same length of your affected limb.

The next thing that you need is something to tie your splint with. You can use obvious materials such as rope, paracord, a belt, or vine, but if these kinds of materials are not available, you can also use strips from clothing, a bandana, or a scarf. Just as long as your tying material is able to secure your splint around your leg it will work, so don't be too picky.

Finally, while it's not necessary, you can also use padding materials so there is at least some comfort in between your limb and the splints themselves. Again, be creative in what you want to use for padding materials.

STEP #2 – PUTTING EVERYTHING INTO POSITION

Before you actually begin tying your splints around your broken limb, you want to put them in place. Lay your tying materials under your limb with roughly an equal length on either side. One of these materials should be near your ankle or wrist, another one below your knee or elbow, and then the last one should be near your waist or shoulder. Never tie directly around your knee or elbow.

Once the tying materials are in position, place your splints on both sides of your limb and over your tying devices.

STEP #3 – TYING THE SPLINT

Once you have everything in their proper position, you can now begin to actually tie your splints around your limb. Start with the ankle or wrist first and then work your way up. Remember to place your padding materials in between your leg and splints first before actually tying them.

Your ties should be fairly snug but you don't want them to be tight enough to the point that they cut off or inhibit blood circulation. That's the last thing that you want to do. To test the snugness of the splints, if you can slide at least two of your fingers next to each other in between the affected limb and the splint, it's perfect. If you can fit less or more fingers in between the limb and the splint, then the splint is too tight or too loose respectively.

STEP #4 – TREATING YOURSELF AFTER THE SPLINT

Earlier in this article, we mentioned that you would also have to apply a dressing to your affected limb if it's an open fracture. If your injury is indeed an open injury, you've probably stopped the bleeding already and applied some form of dressing. Now go back to that dressing and re-evaluate it: you'll want a clean but damp piece of cloth immediately over the wound, followed by a dry piece of clean cloth over it that is secured by either cordage or tape. Make sure that this dressing does not inhibit the splint in anyway.

It's also important that you make sure you do not go into shock during or after applying the splint. Shock is more likely to happen with an open fracture or where the fracture is more serious. Symptoms of shock include rapid but shallow breathing, moist skin, coming into and out of consciousness, blue skin, physical weakness, and a confusion at what is happening.

If you feel that you may be going into shock, lay down flat on your back and get warm by wrapping yourself in a blanket, coat, or a sleeping bag. Control your breathing and stay hydrated.

You won't want to move in the next few days after applying the splint. Get plenty of rest, eat food to keep your energy levels up, and drink lots of water. To prevent the onset of headaches, soak a bandana or piece of cloth in cool water and lay it over your forehead. Check on your splint and on the dressing if the injury is an open fracture. If the wound has healed in the next couple of days, you can decide what you need to do from there.

Chapter Nine – Snake Bite

A snake bite is something that almost everybody fears, and it is this fear that causes many people to stay indoors rather than go out for a hike on a trail. The reality is that your chances of encountering a dangerous snake in North America to begin with are quite low and your chances of being bitten by one significantly lower. But if you or a member of your group are bitten on a hiking trip, it's important to know how to successfully treat a snake bite victim and that's what this article is all about.

The good news is that the vast majority of snake species in North America are not venomous to humans. The venomous snakes that are here in North America bite just under ten thousand people every year, and only around ten or so of those people end up succumbing to the bite. But even though this figure may seem small, it does not mean that you should believe deadly snakes are not a threat to you. A snake's venom may be intended for prey, such as rodents and birds, but if they are provoked or feel threatened by humans they can attack with a life-threatening bite.

HOW TO PREVENT SNAKE BITES

As a general rule of thumb, do not disturb or provoke a snake that you find in the wilderness regardless of whether it is poisonous or not. This advice may seem like something that anybody would take for granted, but it's still something to be reminded of. The snake will act in self-defense is disturbed enough and can leave enough venom to threaten your life.

Hopefully you won't run into any snakes to begin with. You can do this by avoiding habitats that snakes prefer, such as tall grass and underneath large rocks. Wear long pants and boots that go past your ankles for added security.

Still, you should be prepared for a scenario where either you or someone in your group is bitten by a poisonous snake. If you are prepared then you'll know exactly what to do in such a situation and you can likely save somebody's life.

SYMPTOMS OF A SNAKE BITE

The follow are common symptoms of a snake bite:

- Fang Marks
- Swelling Around the Affected Area
- Extreme Pain
- Burning Sensation
- High Fever
- Rapid Heart Rate
- Poor Muscle Coordination
- Blurry Vision/Dizziness
- Convulsions

THE DO'S AND DON'TS OF TREATING A SNKA BITE

The first thing to do when you or someone in your group is bitten by a snake is to call for emergency help immediately so you can receive professional medical aid as soon as possible. If the snake bite is treated properly, the victim will not be left with severe injuries.

But if professional medical help is not in reach, then you'll have to take matters into your own hands. Here are the do's and don'ts of dealing with snake bites.

- The Do's of Handling a Snake Bite

  - Do remove yourself from striking distance of the snake
  - Do keep the victim calm, quiet, and still by having them lay down
  - Do get the heart rate of the victim under control by keeping their bitten limb at or beneath the level of their heart
  - Do remove any jewelry or clothing that restricts blood circulation to the affected area in any way
  - Do keep the movement of the victim to a bare minimal, especially around their affected area
  - Do allow the snake bite to bleed for at least thirty seconds before you treat it
  - Do apply a splint to the broken limb so that the victim will keep movement of the bite area to a minimal, including if they are panicking
  - Do try to identify the snake (if you can) so that you can inform medical professionals; this way, they will more easily know the type of anti-venom to use when you bring the victim to medical help
  - Do apply a bandana soaked in cool water over the victim's head to bring sweating down

- The Don'ts of Handling a Snake Bite

  - Don't try to suck the venom out with your mouth; this is a myth of treating snake bites that is commonly seen in movies and entertainment, but that in reality only endangers the person sucking out the venom
  - Don't wrap a tourniquet over the snake bite wound, as this is another huge myth when it comes to treating snake bites; if you restrict blood flow to the affected area, the venom will begin killing all cells in the area, but if it is allowed to spread the toxin will become diluted and its potency reduced
  - Don't apply a cool bandana or anything similar to the snake bite; doing so will only limit the circulation of blood to the area and could potentially make the venom more deadly if it becomes cool
  - Don't cut near, around, or over the bite marks; doing so only increases the risk of an infection and very likely won't cut out all of the venom
  - Don't try to kill the snake; this is a waste of time and you only run the risk of another member in your group getting bitten
  - Don't flush the snake bite wound with water; you should clean it and remove any debris to prevent infection, but after that simply cover it with a clean dressing

Getting bitten by a snake may be a nightmare for many hikers and outdoor enthusiasts, and it's certainly something that can turn your enjoyable day of hiking out in nature into the direct opposite. But as long as you treat the snake bite the right way, by following the do's and don'ts that we have listed out in this article, the venom can be overcome. That's why referencing the statistic that we pointed out earlier in this article, the overwhelming majority of individuals who are bitten by a snake will survive.

Chapter Ten – Knife and Bullet Wounds

A knife wound is a serious injury and one that demands immediate attention. While any kind of a stabbing can result in bleeding, the sharper the blade the more bleeding there will be. The reason for this is because a dull blade will cause the arteries and the veins to open and close, whereas sharper blades will leave both of these open and cause more blood to pour out. Furthermore, if the blade goes deep enough, it can puncture internal organs and cause internal bleeding that only makes the situation worse. It's for this reason that internal swelling and organ failure are often what kills the victim of a knife attack who goes without treatment.

But the real reason why a knife wound is so deadly is not so much because of the bleeding, which can be stopped, but rather because of the strong possibility of infection. Not only do knife blades tend to be dirty, which is bad when the metal comes into contact with your flesh and blood, but the open wounds also exposes the vessels and arteries to diseases floating around in the air.

A knife stabbing is very unlikely to kill anyone quickly, but the longer it goes without treatment the more at risk the victim will be, regardless of whether you were attacked by someone with a knife or accidentally sliced yourself with your own.

If the stab or slice from the knife is a relatively shallow cut into the flesh, then all you may need to do is to clean the wound and wrap it with a sterile gauze pad or damage. But if the blade went in deeper and punctured an internal organ, then you need professional medical assistance. The following steps are intended as treatment for more serious knife wounds, but are also simply a means to keep the victim alive until professional medical help reaches the scene:

STEP #1 – ASSESS THE VICTIM

As with any first aid application, your first step is to assess the victim. Here are some questions to ask yourself regarding the victim of a knife attack: are there several slashes and stabs on the body or only one? Where are the wounds located? Is clothing obscuring any wounds? Is the bleeding seeping out slowly or is it spurting out rapidly?

Ask the victim if they can feel any wounds on their body that you can't see. It could be that they don't feel enough pain to know of any more wounds, but talking to them is also one way to keep their heart rate under control and reduce the chances of shock.

Once you've assessed the injuries on the person (and in a timely manner), either clean your hands or put on medical gloves and begin the treatment process.

STEP #2 – LEAVE THE KNIFE IN THE BODY

If the knife is sticking out of the person's body, it is a huge mistake to try to remove it. Removing the blade will speed up the bleed and could also cause more blood vessels to be cut. It is also recommended that you keep the blade steady, so either hold it or have someone else do so throughout the treatment process. The blade should only be removed by medical professionals who can quickly provide surgery to fix the problem.

STEP #3 – APPLY PRESSURE TO THE MOST BLEEDING WOUND FIRST

The wound with the most blood should always be your first priority in dealing with knife wounds. If the blood is spurting, it means that an artery has been severed and it requires immediate attention.

If there are several serious wounds with spurting blood, tightly tie a tourniquet above them to cut off the flow of blood. However, if only one serious wound is present, it is better to apply pressure directly on the wound instead of actually cutting off the flow of blood. If you don't have medical gloves on, then there needs to be a physical barrier in between your skin and the victim's wound to prevent the risk of infection. Use a sterile cloth, bandana, gauze pad, or something else along those lines.

STEP #4 – LIFT THE VICTIM'S ARMS OR LEGS

If there is more than one stab/slash wound on the arms, have the victim sit up if they can and lift their arms above their head. This way the flow of blood will be reduced and less blood will exit the wound. If the wounds are present on the legs, have the victim lie down flat on their back and then lift up their legs onto an elevated platform, such as a box, chair, or a large rock.

STEP #5 – CLEAN THE WOUNDS

At this point, the bleeding should be slowing down significantly and in the smaller wounds it should have stopped. With at least some control of the bleeding, you can now begin to clean the wounds. As with before, start with the most serious wounds and then work your way down to the less serious ones.

Examine the wounds closely for any kind of debris or outside material that could be present inside of them, and remove them. The most effective cleansing agent for an open knife wound is at least one tablespoon of salt mixed with at least one cup of warm water. Even though this mixture will cause more pain on the wound, it will cleanse it of bacteria and debris that you can't see.

Inform the victim that what you are about to do will hurt but is necessary to treat the wound. Peroxide or alcohol are fine alternatives to salt, and you can also just use clean water if that's all you have.

STEP #6 – CLOSE THE SMALLER WOUNDS

Once you've cleaned each of the wounds, it's time to close the smaller ones. Yes, this time we want you to start with the smaller wounds first rather than the larger ones. Bandages, gauze pads with tape, cloth with tape or cordage, and duct tape are all examples of materials that you can use to close these wounds. The wounds should be closed off completely so nothing infectious gets inside.

Take note, that you should continually check on the larger wound or wounds while closing the smaller ones and apply pressure on them to slow down or stop the bleeding.

STEP #7 – TEND TO THE LARGER WOUND

If the larger wound has ceased bleeding, then it is safe to close it as with the smaller wounds. However, if the large wound has continued to bleed and shows no sign of letting up, then stuff it with clean rags and cover those rags with tape. You want this tape to be loose so that it doesn't completely bind the wounds like we did with the smaller ones.

STEP #8 – ALLOW THE VICTIM TO REST

Apply a bandana soaked in cool water over the victim's head and have them lie still so they can rest. Make them as comfortable as you can make them. Check up on them regularly and assess the bandages; if one is too tight, you should loosen it so that the blood can circulate better. Ask the victim how they feel and make sure they stay hydrated by drinking plenty of water.

The capability to treat a knife wound is a vital survival skill and one that can save the life of yourself or something you know. Your goal is to keep everybody in your group alive, and now you know how to do it in the event of a knife injury.

BULLET WOUNDS

You now know how to treat a knife wound, but what about bullet wounds? Treating bullet wounds are tricky, because even though the bullet may have entered one area of the body, it likely stopped or exited at a completely different location.

For this reason, there is no universal step-by-step process for treating a gunshot wound. Instead, you have to use different techniques for different areas of the body. In this article, we will cover how to treat gunshot wounds to the head, chest, abdomen, and the limbs.

Something else that's tricky about gunshot wounds is much of the bleeding could be internal. If so, then more advanced training is needed and you need to get the victim to medical professionals as soon as possible. Signs that internal bleeding is happening include rapidly lowering levels of blood pressure, a rapidly increasing pulse, vomiting, and a lowering alertness level.

TREATING GUNSHOT WOUNDS TO THE HEAD

The biggest factor that you need to take into the most consideration when treating a gunshot wound to the head is the victim's airway, and specifically that there is no blood running down it that could possibly choke them. Keep as much direct pressure on the wound itself, rather than applying a tourniquet around or above it. You'll want to apply slightly less pressure to the wound if you believe the bullet has cut an artery.

If the victim is conscious, then have them sit up and lean in a forward direction. If the victim is not conscious, then turn them around on their side and bend their knee forward. Both of these measures will reduce the flow of blood to the head and help stop the bleeding.

Once you've applied pressure to the wound and turned the victim around or have them sit up to reduce the flow of bleeding, you can then treat the wound with a dressing. The best type of dressing for a gunshot wound is called an occlusive dressing, which is defined as a water-tight and air-tight dressing that is designed to completely seal the wound. It can be made out of something as simple as plastic wrap, a bandana, or a gauze pad. Apply the dressing to the wound so that it is completely sealed.

TREATING GUNSHOT WOUNDS TO THE CHEST

The factors unique to a gunshot wound in the chest is injury that's been dealt to the spine and how much air the victim is taking in. For the latter reason, the occlusive dressing is going to be slightly different than the one you applied to the head.

First though, let's talk about the spine. The spine is located in the back part of the chest, so you'll want the victim to be entirely still throughout the treatment process so that no further damage is dealt to the spinal cord if the victim has been already damaged there. However, if the lungs, heart, or the spine have been directly hit, then there is little that you can do on your own other than try to find professional medical help.

When applying the occlusive dressing to the gunshot wound in the chest, you have to simultaneously prevent more air from getting in while allowing the extra air inside to get out. Lay down plastic wrap on the wound over the chest, and then when the diaphragm sucks in the air, the plastic wrap will become a vacuum that in turn sucks the object inside of the wound. When the air escapes the chest, it can easily push the plastic wrap upwards. Keep in mind this is only a temporary solution until professional medical help arrive; doctors will likely use a chest tube to treat a gunshot wound to the chest.

TREATING A GUNSHOT WOUND TO THE ABDOMEN

The biggest factor unique to a gunshot wound to the abdomen is the risk of organ injury. If the bullet wound is open enough, you might be able to see the intestines inside. Apply a clean but moist dressing over this part of the wound; the purpose of this is to protect the organs inside and prevent them from falling out.

However, if the intestines have been directly hit or are ripped open, then the victim needs urgent medical care. Even if you manage to stop the bleeding, they can still die of an infection that sets in.

Last but not least, DO NOT allow a victim of a gunshot wound to the abdomen to intake any food or water, at least not until much of the pain has subsided. This will be hard, since the victim may be extremely thirsty, but remember that it's important so that the organs don't worsen. If you do permit the patient to have any water, only allow them to drink a little bit at long intervals. When professional medical help arrives, they'll insert IV's in the patient to get fluids into them.

TREATING A GUNSHOT WOUND TO THE LIMBS

A factor unique to a gunshot wound to the limbs is that the wounded limb must be elevated above the heart level of the patient. Have them lie down on their back, and then elevate their wounded limb while keep all other limbs flat on the ground.

Then, apply pressure to the gunshot wound with your fingers while you wrap a pressure bandage around it. If the bleeding continues, wrap a tourniquet above the wound. If a bone has been hit, treat the wound like you would a fractured limb and make a pair of splints for the patient.

If the gunshot wound still won't stop bleeding even after you've applied direct pressure, wrapped a pressure bandage, and tied a tourniquet, then you'll need to apply direct pressure to the brachial artery if the wound is in the arm or the femoral artery if it's in the leg. The brachial artery is located on the inner arm below the armpit, while the femoral artery is located between the front part of the leg and the hip.

Chapter Eleven – Carrying an Injured Person

If you are in a survival situation or a disaster scenario, and a member of your group goes down with an injury that is bad enough that they cannot walk on their own, you may be faced with the task of carrying them out to safety.

Without a shadow of a doubt, the first thing that you need to do is assess the person's injuries and give them first aid while keeping them as comfortable as possible. However, if the person's injuries do not heal soon, you will be faced with a critical decision to make: do you leave the wounded person there with some provisions and then go out for help on your own, or do you try to carry them out yourself?

This chapter will tell you what to do if you determine, to the best of your ability, that the best course of action to take is to carry out or drag the person yourself. There are many different methods you can use to carry an injured individual from place to place, and we'll cover a few of these methods in a moment. But first, let's discuss when you absolutely should NOT carry a wounded person out.

WHEN NOT TO CARRY OR DRAG A WOUNDED PERSON OUT

It's always a bad idea to try and carry someone out if he or she has suffered a spinal injury, especially if the injury is severe. Trying to carry someone with a spinal injury can dramatically increase both the pain and the damage of the injury, and if gone far enough, can potentially even cause them to become paralyzed. You want to avoid this from happening at all costs.

You can generally tell if someone has sustained a spinal injury if they are unable to move their neck, are informing you of extreme pain in their neck or their back, if their neck or head is twisted in any way, if they experience pain when flexing their limbs, or if they are experiencing paralysis or numbness in their limbs.

If someone in your group has suffered a spinal injury, stabilize them rather them out. Place cushions (made out of whatever resources you have) on both sides of their head so it won't roll, use the jaw thrust method for opening their airway if they are experiencing difficulty breathing, and don't take off their helmet if they were wearing one at the time of the injury (doing so can only make the spine worse).

With that being said, let's examine some of the different methods you can use for carrying a wounded person out to safety if they haven't suffered a spinal injury and if you feel, under your circumstances, that it's a better option than leaving them with provisions and searching for help on your own.

METHOD #1 – FIREMAN'S CARRY

As the name suggests, this method of carrying a wounded person is the same one that is used by firefighters. Considering the fact that firefighters constantly find themselves involved in very complex situations and need to get people out to safety quick, it wouldn't exactly be wise to hold the methods they use in low regard.

To use the fireman's carry method, following these steps:

1. Bring the person up to their feet and hold them from behind their waist so that you are looking at them face to face; your dominant hand should be the one holding them

2. Using your other hand, grab the person by their wrist on the same side and raise their arm over their head

3. Squat down and position your knee on the side of your dominant hand between the person's leg

4. Start to heft the person over your shoulders

5. While lifting the person, bring your arm to around their thighs and shift the weight of the person over your shoulders

6. Slowly stand while keeping your back as straight as it can be; you want your legs to be your primary source of lifting power

The firemen's carry method is an effective way to lift and carry someone to safety, but it's also best used for short term endeavors because it requires a lot of exertion on your part especially.

A safer method than actually lifting a person is to drag them. Lifting a person not only puts more weight on you, but it also means that the injured person runs the risk of falling off and becoming even more injured.

When dragging a person, you will want to keep them in a straight line so that their spine will not twist. There are three ways to drag someone: the clothing drag, the leg drag, or the arm drag method.

CLOTHING DRAG

The clothing drag method is best used if the person has injuries on both their arms and legs. The best place on the clothing to grab is underneath the armpits, because this is the least likely place for the clothing to tear when being dragged and it also keeps the injured person's head above the ground. Always bend your knees and utilize your weight by leaning back when dragging someone.

LEG DRAG

The leg drag method should be only used when a person hasn't sustained any leg injuries, but still cannot walk on their own. Your want your back to remain as straight as possible while dragging them, and the best way to do this is by grabbing them by their ankles. Then lean back and slowly drag the person away.

ARM DRAG

When a person has leg injuries, you should always use the arm drag method in place of the leg drag. Bend your knees and ensure that your back is kept straight when dragging the person. You can squeeze the elbows of the injured person against their head so that it does not drag. Again, you can use your own weight by leaning back and moving slowly to drag them away to safety.

Chapter Twelve – Medicinal Plants for First Aid

Today, we've gotten pretty used to modern medication and technologies to ward off against diseases, infections, and physical injuries. You might be asking yourself how people were able to care for their injuries and infections before the advent of the modern medications of today, and the answer is in plants that contain strong medicinal properties. In fact, you very likely drive or walk by medicinal plants each day.

In a survival situation, medicinal plants can be a true lifesaver. But it only works if you can positively identify the plant in the first place and then know how to prepare and administer it. In this article, we'll run down eleven different medicinal plants that commonly grow in North America, and learn the visual characteristics and medicinal properties of each one.

In alphabetical order:

BIRCH BARK

As the name suggests, birch bark grows on birch trees. Not only does scraped birch bark work beautifully as a natural tea, but it's quite the efficient painkiller as well. The general recommended daily dosage of birch bark is a maximum of one hundred and twenty milligrams a day; any higher dosages than that can potentially cause a hurting stomach and nausea, so be careful. The best way to prepare birch bark is by mixing a small portion of it in water and then boiling it for ten to fifteen minutes. The resulting mixture doubles as a tea and as a painkiller!

BLACKBERRY LEAVES

Almost everyone should agree that blackberries are extremely tasty, but not nearly everyone knows of the medicinal properties the leaves contain. The fact is that blackberry leaves are one of the best natural treatments for diarrhea. Mix at least an ounce of a fresh leaf with a cup of hot water, and blend it together like you would a tea.

BURDOCK

Burdock was originally native to the Eastern Hemisphere before it was introduced to North America many years ago, where it has thrived ever since. You can identify burdock, which is also known as Arctium, by its purple leaf stocks that are longer than the leaves themselves, and white and purple flower heads with stiff prickles surrounding him. The leaves and roots of burdock can help purify the blood in your body when consumed. Boil the roots and fresh leaves in water before removing the roots and fresh leaves and eating them; the boiling water not only cleanses the plant, but it removes much of the rather bitter taste too.

DANDELIONS

We see dandelions literally everyday around town, and while they may be nothing more than an annoying weed in our daily life, in a survival situation the roots can improve digestion in the body and also serve as a liver stimulant. Mix a tablespoon of the root in a bowl of hot water before consuming.

ECHINACEA

An herb native to eastern and central North America, Echinacea is noted for its tall stems that can exceed four feet in total height, purple and/or pink flowers, and a brown central cone. Native Americans historically have used the roots and leaves of Echinacea as a treatment for the common cold for hundreds of years. Mix them in hot water as a tea.

ELDERBERRY

The well known and commonplace elderberry plant is easily one of the most versatile medicinal plants on this list. When it is applied directly to the skin, there are few plants that are as efficient for treating open wounds as the elderberry. When taken orally, it can treat common colds and respiratory problems. When ingested nasally, elderberries can reduce sinus infections and swelling inside the mucous membranes. Just think of all of the jam that you can make out of elderberries and then how you can double that jam as part of your medicinal stockpile. The only concern with the elderberry is that the actual berries themselves are a little toxic when raw, so you'll want to boil them for at least fifteen to twenty minutes.

LAVENDER

Most of us are probably familiar with lavender as a fragrance, but throughout history it has been used as a treatment for skin burns and bug bites. Simply crush a few leaves and apply them directly to the skin. To use as a medicinal oil, fill up a jar with the leaves and then combine them with some olive oil. Allow this mixture to soak for up to two months, and you have fresh medicinal oil that you can use for skin issues. Lavender should not be used by small children or women who are pregnant.

LEMON BALM

You can include bruised lemon balm leaves in your lemonade to make it more tasty. More importantly, you can use the tea from lemon balm as a cold sore remedy. So effective is lemon balm at this that many current prescription medications for cold sores include lemon balm as one of their primary ingredients.

PLANTAIN

This oval shaped plant with green flowers and dense, spiked stamens is originally native to Europe and Asia, but was introduced to North America many years ago and continues to thrive here. You'll find plantain in many lawns and yards throughout the United States. But what good does plantain do as a medicine? The answer is it's one of nature's best treatments for bee, wasp, and scorpion stings. All you need to do is crush some of the leaves into smaller pieces and mix it with a little water to form a paste. Apply the paste directly to the wound and wait for it to dry off, and pain relief from the sting will follow.

YARROW

Yarrow is a perennial herb that belongs in any medicinal garden. The leaves of the yarrow are great for treating open wounds and abrasions on the skin because they can stop the bleeding and protect against infections. Simply crush the dried leaves and mix with a little water before applying directly to the wounded area.

This is just a small handful of the many different medicinal plants that are out there. It would definitely be a good idea to contain a small book of medicinal plants in your survival kit so you can positively identify them when in an actual survival situation. You never know, but it could be a humble weed or herb that saves your life by warding off an infection or eliminating a respiratory problem.

CONCLUSION

Congratulations on reading this book! I hope that you were able to find the information you were looking for on giving first aid in a survival situation, so that you will be able to save your or someone else's life in a time where you're away from civilization and you only have natural resources at your disposal.

First aid in general has to be one of your biggest priorities in any survival situation. Knowing and applying the first aid skills that we have covered in this book could mean the difference between life and death should ever sustain a life threatening injury.

Good luck!

THANK YOU FOR READING!

YOU CAN CHECK OUT MY OTHER E-BOOKS BY **CLICKING BELOW**

AMAZON AUTHOR PAGE

If you enjoyed this e-book, then please share your thoughts by leaving a review on Amazon!

Made in the USA
Coppell, TX
09 September 2022

82902349R00026